Praise for

"Since the Winnicotts tried to describe the real essence of proper care of children suffering with war-related loss and trauma in London hostels in the early 1940's, we've been resisting the idea that *holding* is the most important thing of all. Sarah Dickey helps us to calm ourselves, step aside from all the clinical and development arguments, and be reminded of what is at the heart of it all.

So many questions asked by teachers, foster parents and all those who give care to children and to their parents would be answered immediately if we just learned to inquire, as Sarah Dickey does: "How would you like to be held?"

Haunting photographs, combined with a purposeful-ly-minimum number of words: Who would imagine that this could be the recipe for communicating one of the most complicated but essentially simple needs of all humans: to be *held*? Sarah Dickey grabs us and won't let us go."

—Michael Trout, Director of the Infant-Parent Institute

"Holding and touch are a vital part of our human experience. Sarah's book reminds us to be intentional in holding our babes through every stage of life. The world will be better if we take her words and turn them into conscious actions."

—Robbie Davis Floyd, author of *Birth as an American Rite of Passage*

"This book is a nest, a home, an embrace, a full breath. This book is a tangible hug, a prayer, a loving home. It is bursting with wisdom, beauty and compassion. You will feel infinitely calmer and richer for having read this book. And yes, you will feel HELD."

—Heidi Rose Robbins, The Radiance Project Podcast and author of *Wild Compassion*

"Every human being needs a conscious loving embrace, to be held and to hold. This holding is essential for regulating the nervous system, body temperature and heart rate, mental and emotional stability, and spiritual connection. When we feel held by our parents, by others, and by ourselves, then we can settle into and have greater confidence and accomplishment in our lives.

"Consciously holding with love, with touch, with our words, with our song, with our every breath, instills human wisdom and knowing, from the very beginning and at any stage of our human development, that we are deeply loved and supported — truly held while embarking on our life's journey.

"Sarah L. Dickey invites us to inquire into how we each want to be held. The conscious art of embracing is a golden key to living a connected and love filled life. A must read for everyone!"

—Nina Ketscher, Founder Your Soul's Spark,
Holistic Integrative Therapist

Other Books by Sarah L. Dickey

Ode to Love: A Journey of Awakening

Sweetly Speaking: Living an Inspired Life

Seasons: 31 Heart Offerings

Holding

Holding

The CONSCIOUS ART of EMBRACING

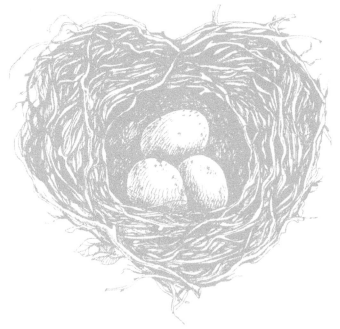

Sarah L. Dickey

Pre & Perinatal Psychology Educator

Cool Creative Press

Holding
The Conscious Art of Embracing

COOL CREATIVE PRESS
PO Box 5370
Poland, OH 44514
www.sarahldickey.com

Publisher's Cataloging-In-Publication Data
(Prepared by The Donohue Group, Inc.)

Names: Dickey, Sarah L., author.
Title: Holding : the conscious art of embracing / Sarah L. Dickey, Pre & Perinatal Psychology Educator.
Description: Lisbon, Ohio : Cool Creative Press, [2021]
Identifiers: ISBN 9780999072042 (paperback w/ french flaps)
Subjects: LCSH: Love, Maternal. | Parent and child. | Touch--Psychological aspects. | Hugging. | Mind and body. | BISAC: HEALTH & FITNESS / Pregnancy & Childbirth. | BODY, MIND & SPIRIT / Inspiration & Personal Growth. | SELF-HELP / Personal Growth / Happiness.
Classification: LCC HQ755.83 .D53 2021 | DDC 306.874--dc23

Library of Congress Control Number: 2021903505

ISBN Number: 978-0-9990720-4-2

Printed in the USA

Editor: Gail M. Kearns, www.topressandbeyond.com
Copy Editor: Cindy Conger, JustWrite Communications
Book and cover design: *the*BookDesigners
Cool Creative Press logo designed by Starr Struck Studio

This book is dedicated to all hearts.
May we unearth with compassion our need
to be held in a multitude of ways.

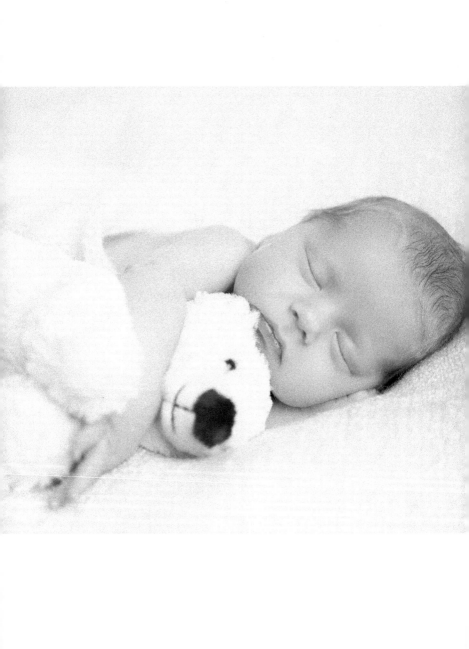

Gratitude Notes

Gratitude to my ever-present-in-the-moment middle nephew for his delight in being held.

Gratitude to Robin Grille for his work and how my time studying with him awoke a deep need to be held. Through his inner child process, I discovered within the walls of my being that I continue to have what he names a deep "psycho-emotional developmental need" from my own perinatal period. As an adult, I have a capacity to cultivate his antidote—a restorative, healing developmental nutrient. And it has been life changing, because, as Robin suggested in my time with him, "These needs aren't of the past, we continue to have the flavor throughout our lives."

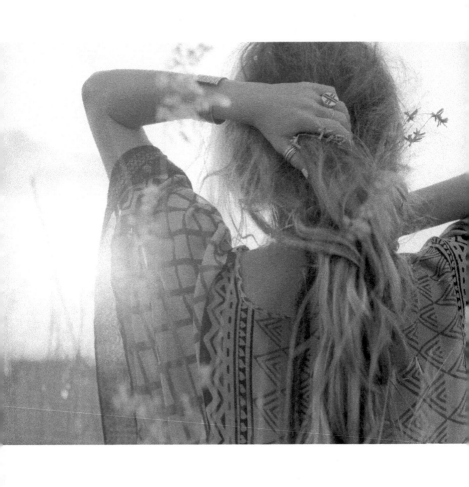

Dear Friends,

This book was a "waking up" for me of a need that lives deeply within my life, decades away from my birth. As Robin Grille encouraged in his teachings, holding is essential for our successful evolution and advancement. As my sweet lover-of-life nephew reminds me, holding is continually emerging.

The sweetness of holding myself in a new way has brought more love and coherence to my life.

I hope this book embraces you and your little one; that it fosters a deep sense of loving kindness. I like to think of holding as a muscle that we work every day of our lives. We create a tradition of holding long before our child comes to us.

As I was inspired by this notion of holding, I observed holding myself in new ways. I found a stillness that my body, mind, and spirit could relax into. I found myself leaning into invisible realms and feeling the benevolence of wonder, the spark of curiosity.

I wonder how this tree might hold me?

I wonder how I can be in relationship with

those I love from afar.

How can I hold them even now?

I invite you to hold yourselves in unfamiliar ways. I implore you to pioneer new possibilities and carve out deep territories of compassion within your hearts. It is my aspiration that this book stirs you to hold yourself, those you love, and the whole world in new ways.

Sarah

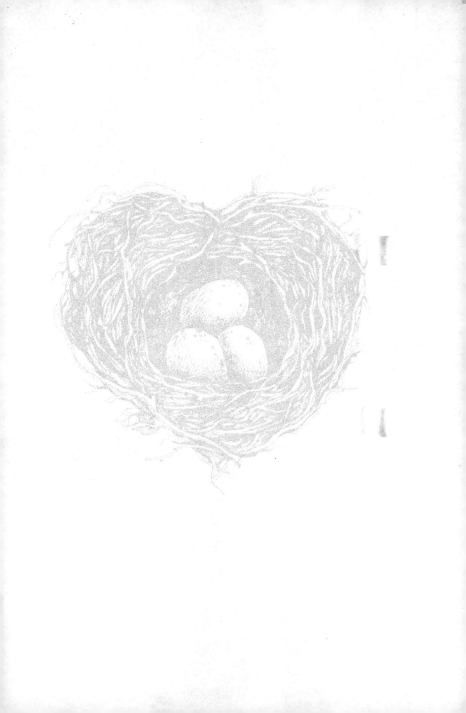

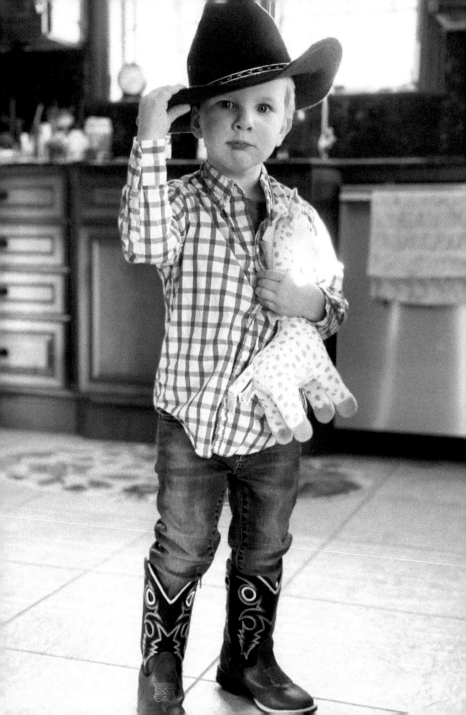

An Invitation

During 2020, I heard from so many that they miss holding one another, miss being in physical connection with community. My nephew reminds me that this need is with us from the very beginning. If I close my eyes, I can feel him greeting me. Jumping out of my car, I can hear his tiny voice approaching me with shouts of Shay-Shay (a tender name he has given to me). As he comes barreling toward me, we meet each other with joy. "Hold me Shay-Shay, hold me."

His stature is framed with love. His eyes as deep as the bluest ocean. His little crooked grin pulsates out ahead of him. He radiates curiosity and is well-versed in wonder. The Earth and backhoes offer his playful spirit sheer delight. He snuggles with blankies as he grows into his independence. He is a gift from the great beyond. He, and his siblings, have rocked my heart wide open. Their presence wakes up a deep ocean of love in my heart.

As I scoop him up, I am reminded of how much love I have for this sweet boy. He looks at me and says, "Put me down Shay-Shay. Come and play with me." Hand in hand we run off toward the next adventure. Play is a deep way of holding. Awareness is a deep way of holding. Presence is a deep way of holding.

In holding him, I meet within myself a deep need to be held. An ache of sorts to notice the ways that holding might occur. As the year unfolded and the physical holding became less frequent, I took a class with world-renowned psychologist Robin Grille. He has more than thirty years of clinical experience and is the author of *Parenting for a Peaceful World* and *Heart-to-Heart-Parenting*.

Robin's work inspired many of the thoughts on these pages. Through his teaching, I came to an awareness that my need to be held is very appropriate and promotes long-standing emotional intelligence. Robin suggests the developmental need of being held begins in-utero. He helped me to realize that this need spans our lifetime, and even if we missed it at the beginning, it can be repaired and restored at any age.

As I touch this need in my life, I recognize a universal longing for all of us to hold and be held. As I am greeted by my young nephews and niece, they remind me that holding can occur in a multitude of ways. We can hold with our arms. We can hold with our words. We can hold with our very presence.

Please note that when I call forth the mommas on these pages, I call forth all who identify as male, female, or non-binary, who hold with maternal tenderness.

I invite you to consciously embrace your babes, here and not yet conceived, and yourself. My heart longs to make a difference for all the children of our world, and all the adults who have an inner child longing to be held.

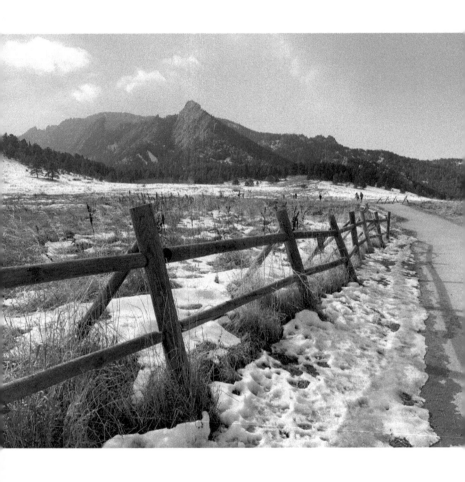

Holding During Pre-Conception

Pre-conception is the time before physical form takes shape.
Imagine standing at the base of a mountain, trusting that
you will be equipped and able to meet the journey ahead of
you. There will be moments of movement, and there will
be moments of pause. During this time of waiting, perhaps
there are great surges of love in anticipation of your little
one's arrival. Perhaps you touch a deep tenderness within
your heart to become a parent, an ache within your bones.
Pre-conception offers the fertile space to welcome the soul
who will one day become your child. Maybe there are
words, or possibly deep wordless spaces of love. May you
echo these sentiments internally or aloud.

WE HOLD YOU IN OUR HEARTS.

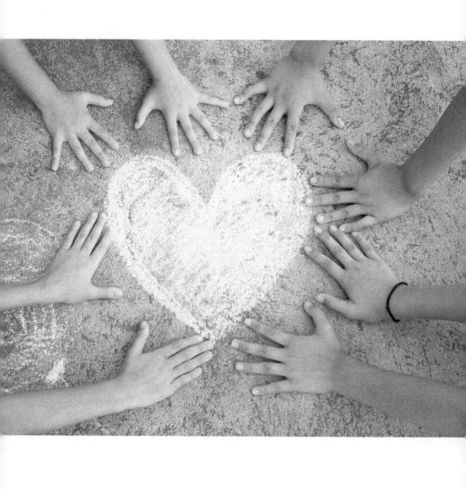

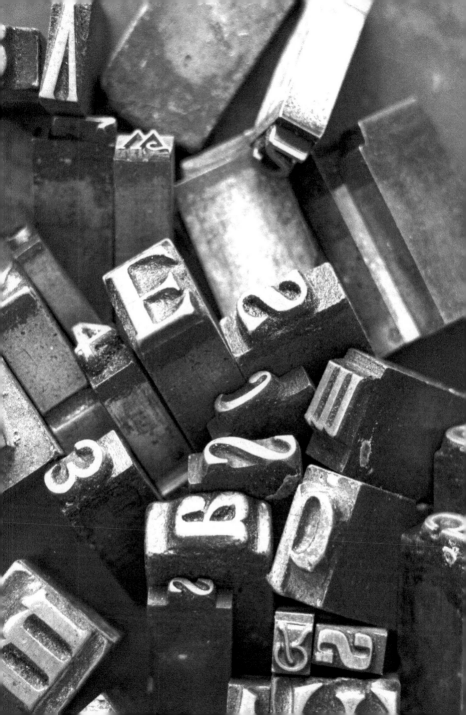

WE HOLD YOU
WITH OUR WORDS.

WE HOLD YOU
IN OUR AWARENESS.

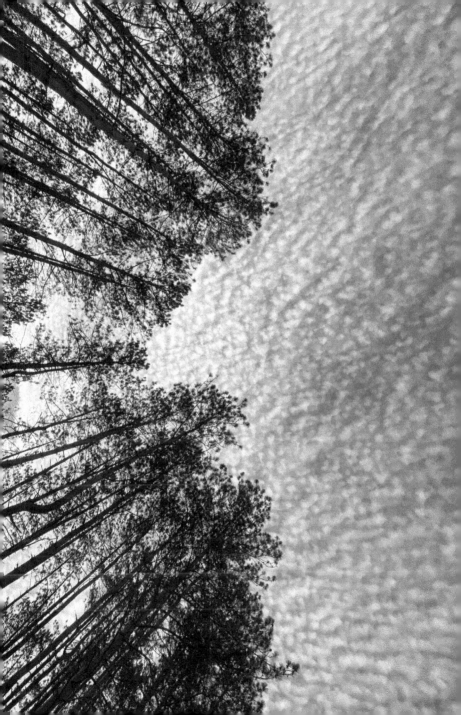

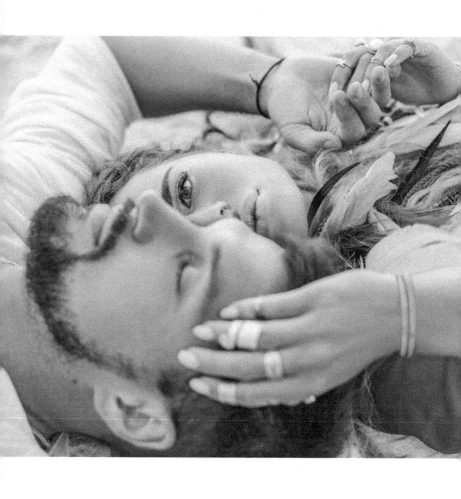

WE HOLD YOU
IN THE STILLNESS.

WE HOLD YOU
IN OUR LOVE MAKING.

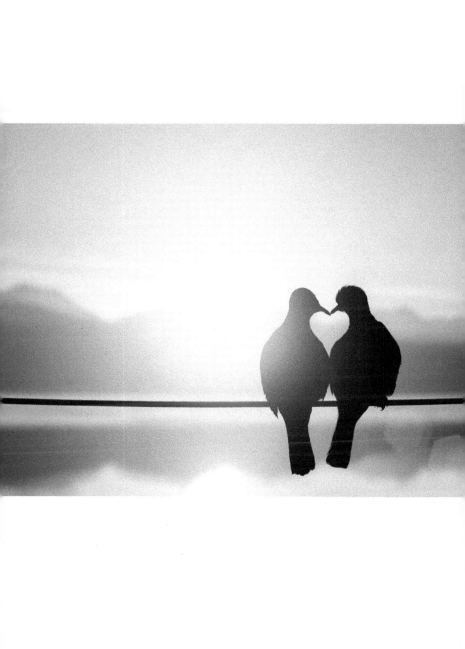

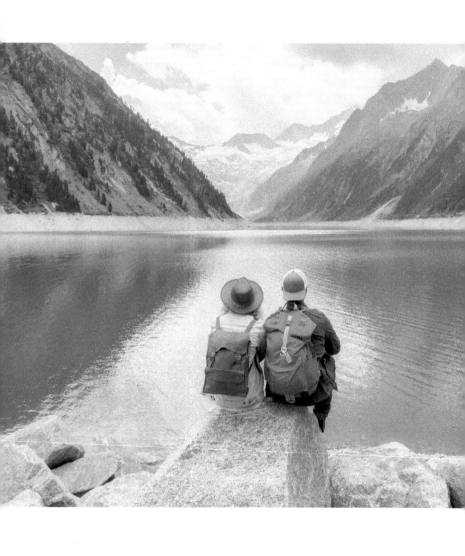

WE HOLD YOU IN OUR THOUGHTS.

WE HOLD YOU
IN OUR HEALING.

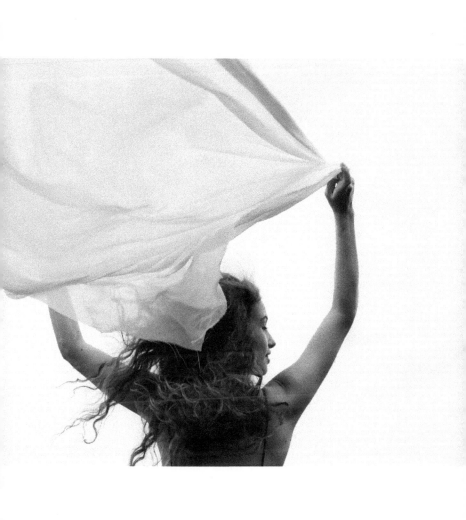

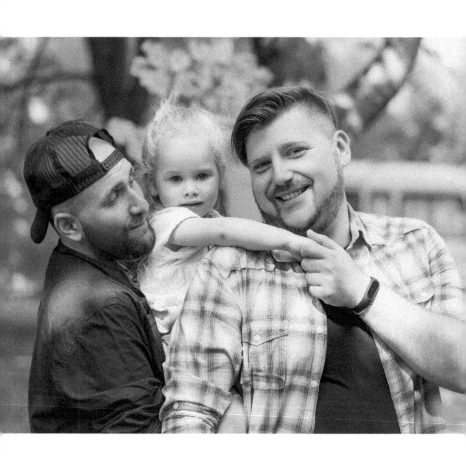

WE HOLD YOU
IN OUR INTENTIONALITY.

WE HOLD YOU
IN OUR PRAYERS.

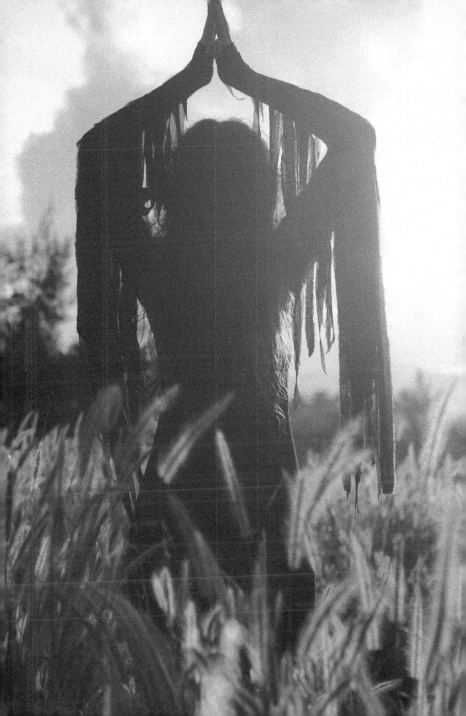

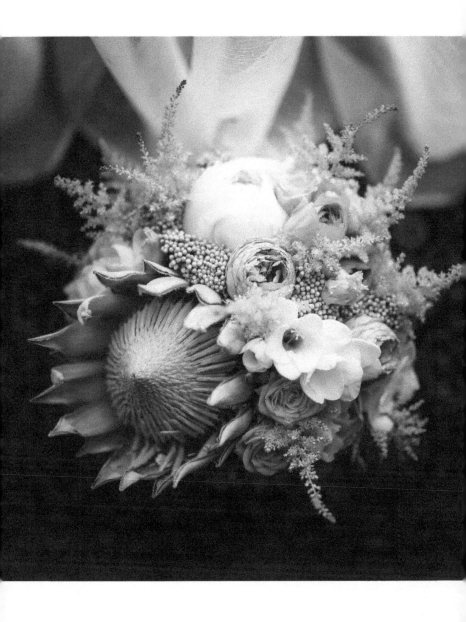

WE HOLD YOU
IN THE ANTICIPATION
OF SPRING BLOSSOMS.

WE HOLD YOU
IN THE LIFE-GIVING
HEAT OF SUMMER.

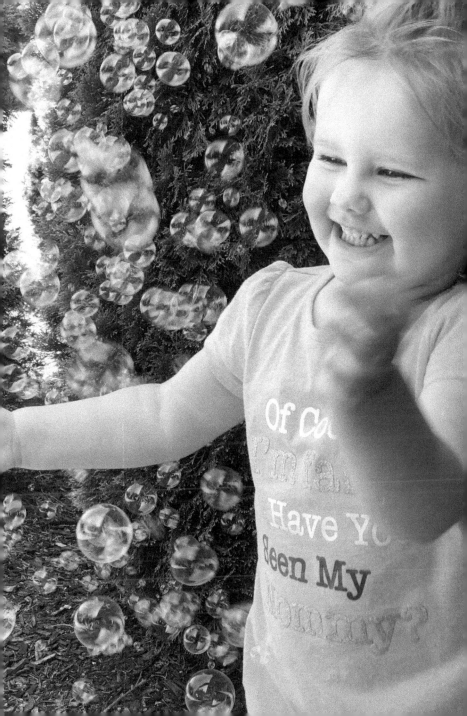

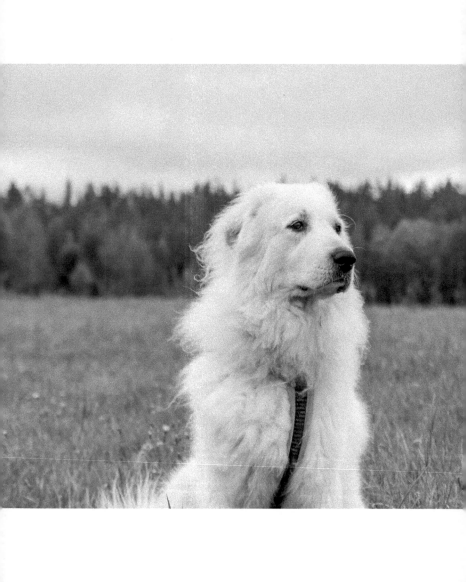

WE HOLD YOU
IN THE TENDER
LETTING GO OF FALL.

WE HOLD YOU
IN THE DEEP
HIBERNATION OF WINTER.

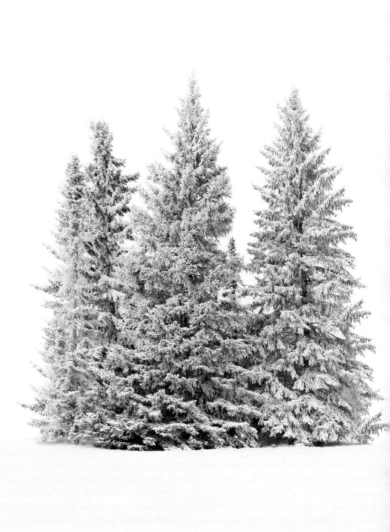

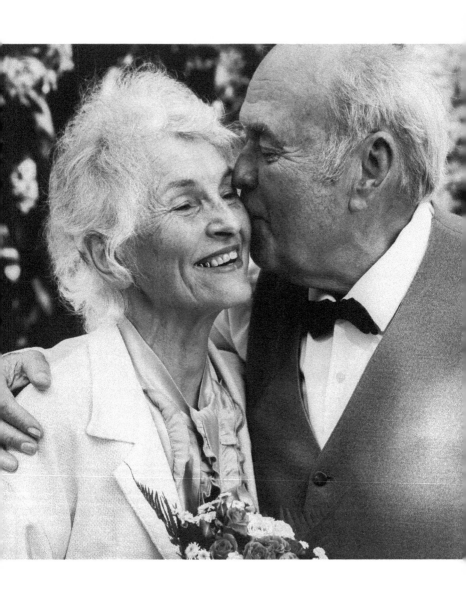

WE HOLD YOU
IN ALL SEASONS
OF OUR LIVES.

WE HOLD YOU IN AN INVISIBLE WORDLESS SPACE.

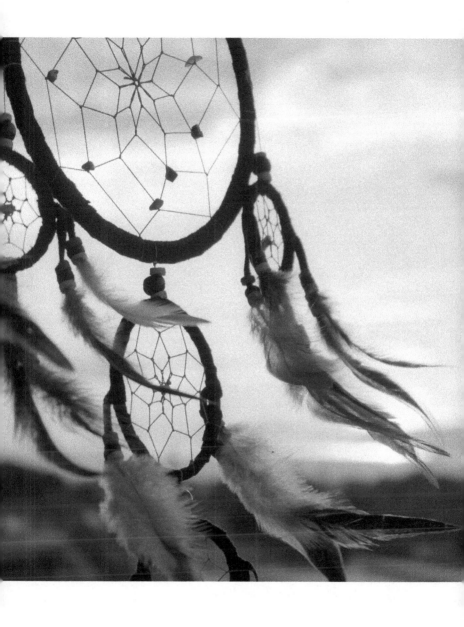

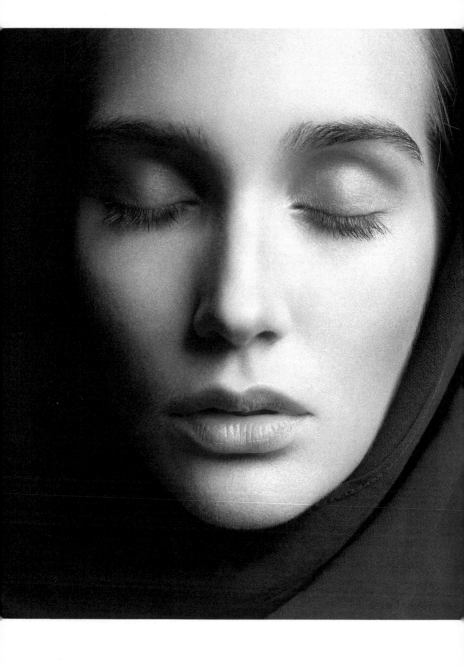

WE HOLD YOU
IN HUMILITY.

WE HOLD YOU IN SACREDNESS.

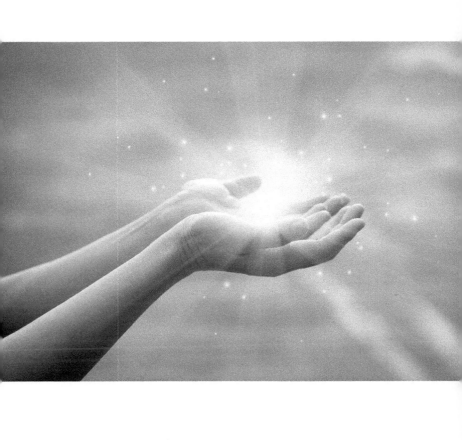

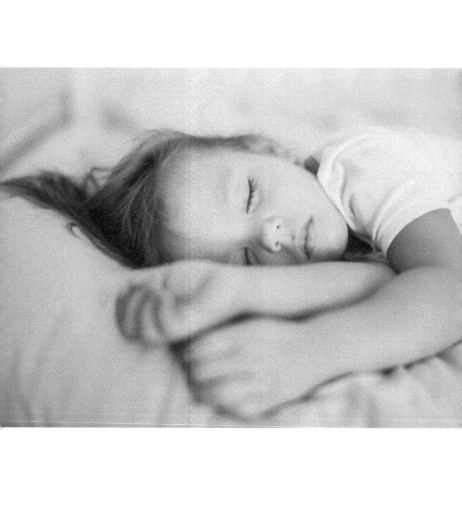

WE HOLD YOU
IN SAFETY.

WE HOLD YOU
IN CONSCIOUSNESS.

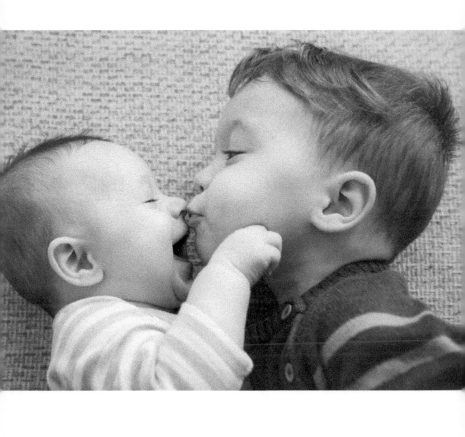

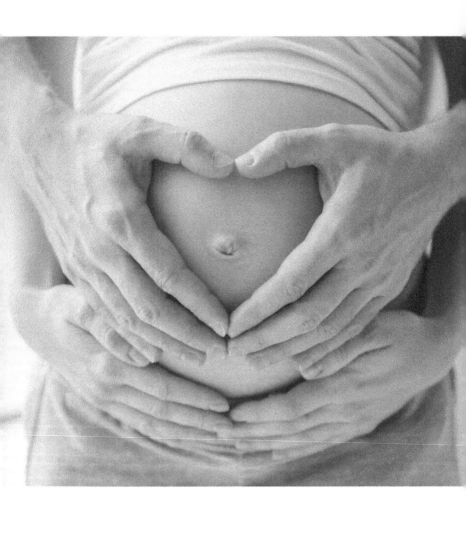

Holding During Gestation

Did you know that by four months in utero your child's hearing is developed? I invite you to create a space to connect with your little one. I hope you feel a deep invitation to read these words to your baby. Create a space—a sacred pause in your daily routine—to drop into stillness with him or her. What do you notice in this space with each other? I hope you feel the freedom to add whatever else you might be wishing to express to your little one. Let it pour from your heart like a gentle stream flowing down the mountain.

YOUR CHILD
CAN HEAR YOU.

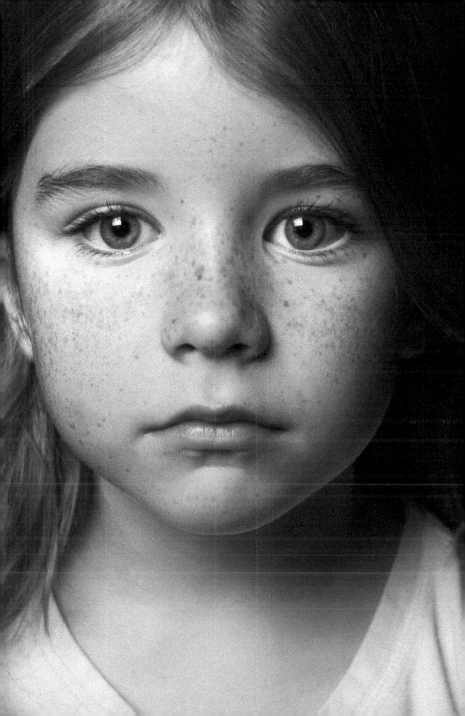

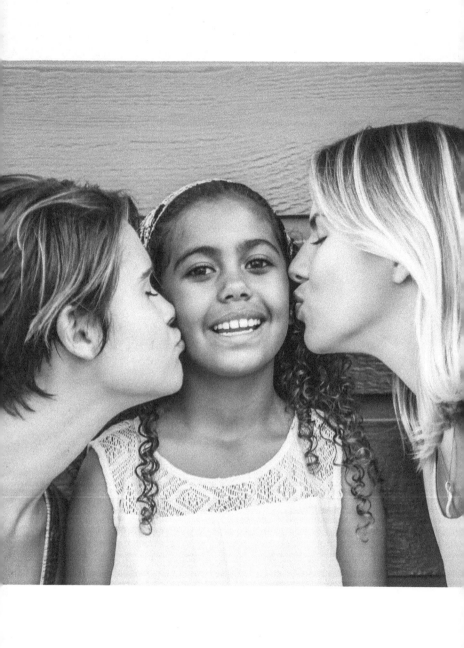

YOUR CHILD
CAN FEEL YOU.

YOUR CHILD IS DEEPLY LISTENING.

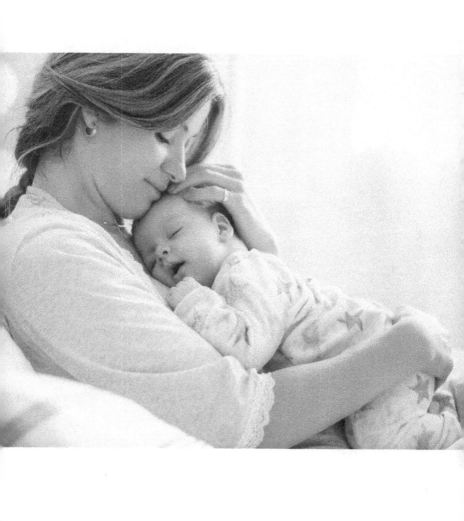

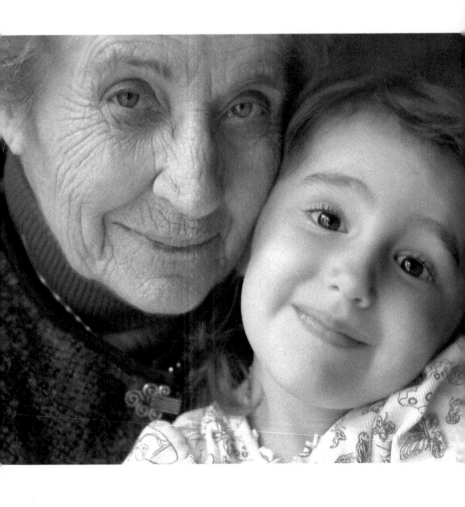

WE ASK OUR
HEALED RADIANT
ANCESTORS TO HOLD YOU.

WE ASK THE EARTH
TO HOLD THE BLESSING
OF YOU.

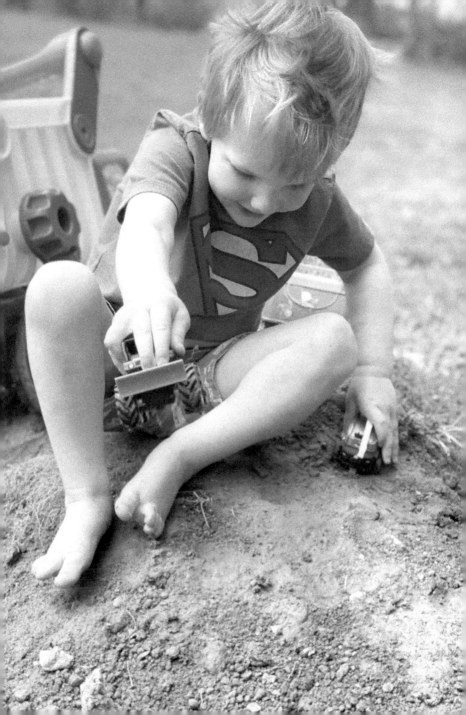

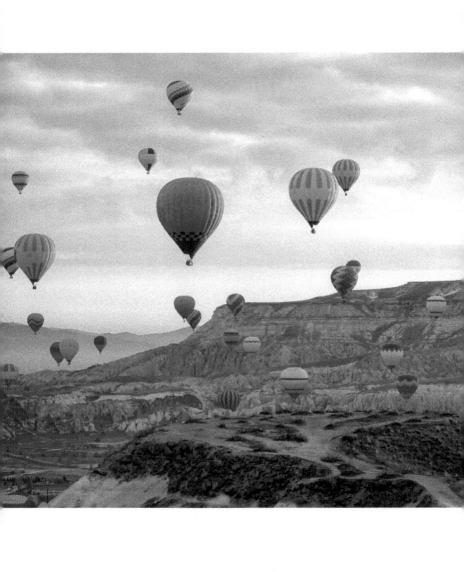

WE ASK THE SKY
TO HOLD THE VASTNESS
OF YOUR PRESENCE.

WE ASK THE WINDS
TO HOLD THE CAPTIVATING
ENERGY THAT IS YOU.

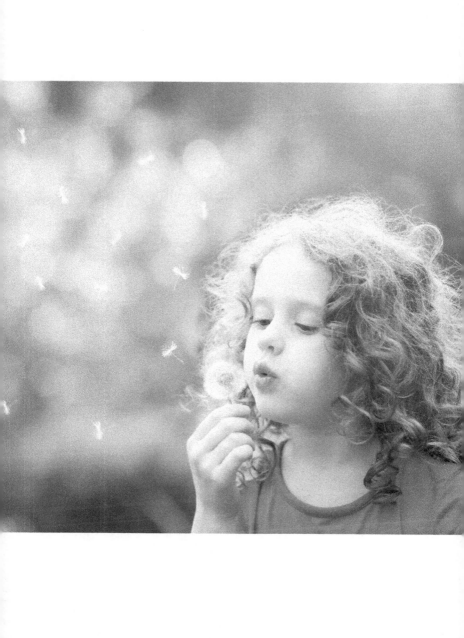

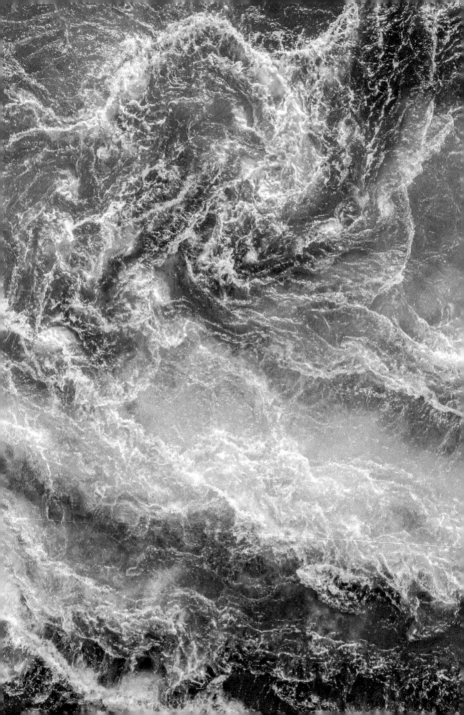

WE ASK THE RAINS
TO HOLD AND CLEANSE YOU.

WE ASK THE SUN
TO HOLD THE RADIANCE
OF YOU.

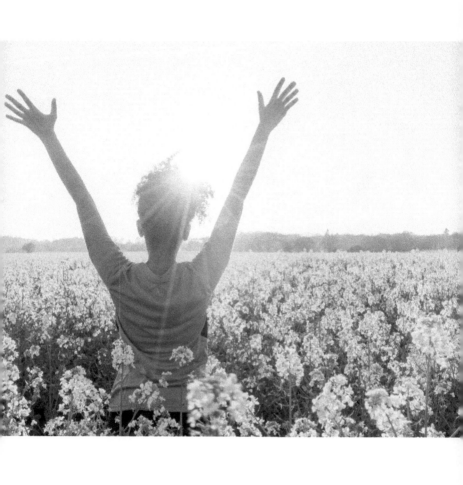

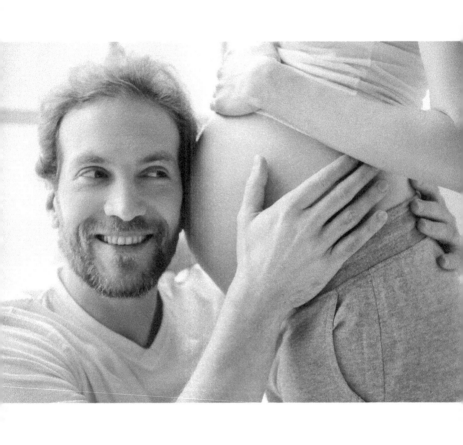

WE ASK THE WALLS
OF YOUR MOTHER'S BODY
TO HOLD YOU.

WE ASK OUR
LOVE TO HOLD YOU.

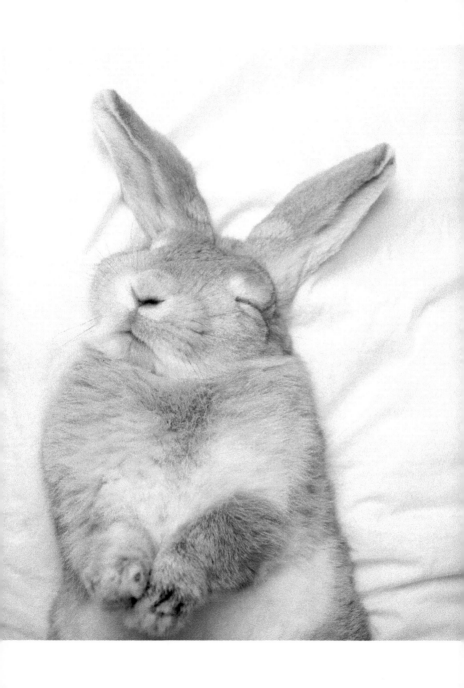

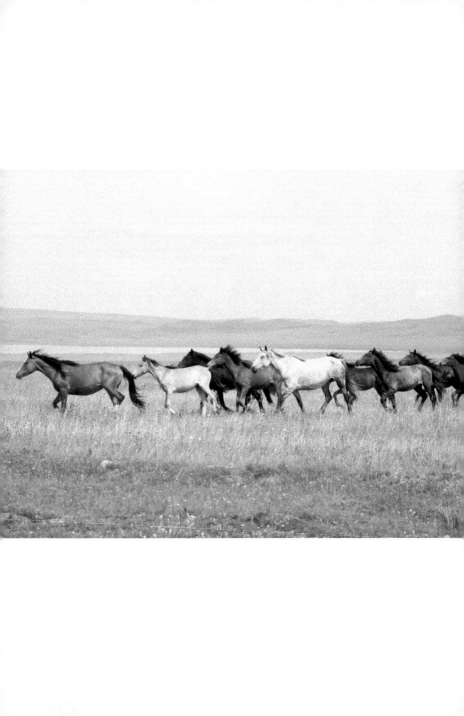

WE ASK OUR
FRIENDS TO HOLD YOU.

WE ASK OUR VOICES
TO HOLD YOU.

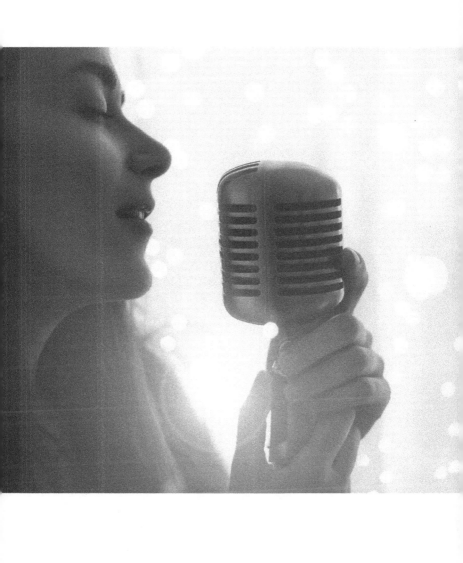

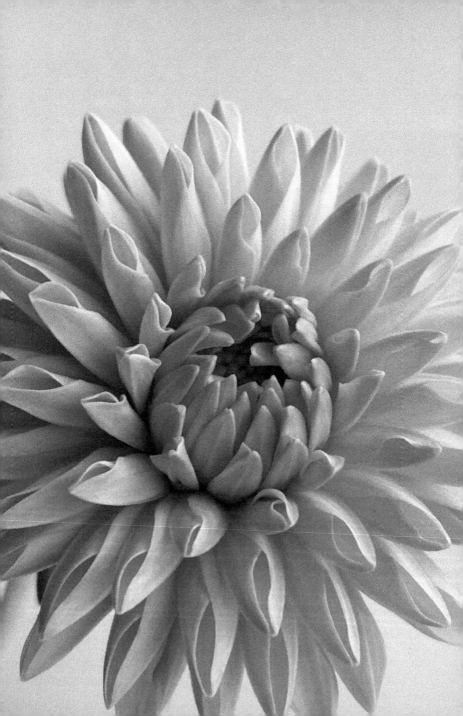

WE ASK THE VAST STILLNESS
OF LIFE TO HOLD YOU.

WE ASK OUR GENTLE TOUCH TO HOLD YOU.

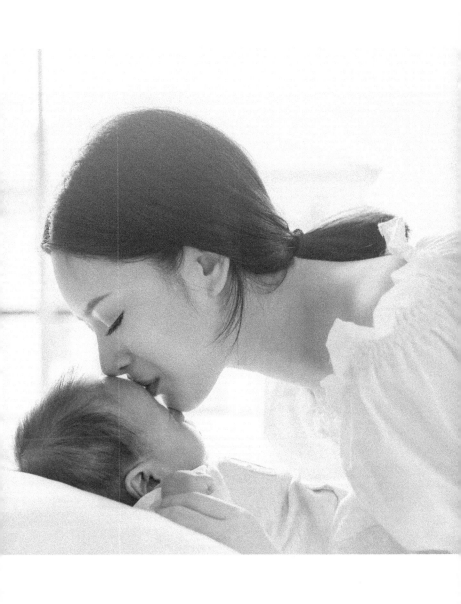

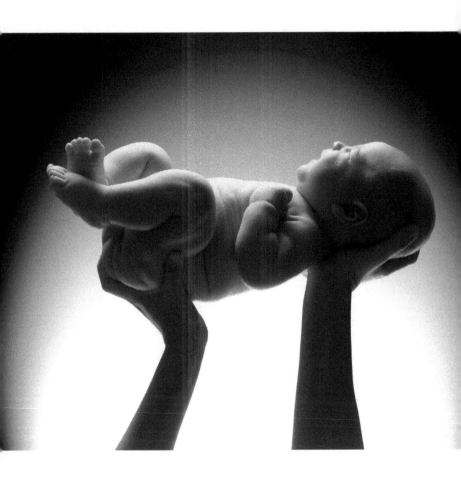

WE ASK THE WALLS
OF THE BIRTH CENTER OR
HOSPITAL TO HOLD YOU.

WE ASK THE DOCTORS,
NURSES, DOULAS, MIDWIVES
AND OTHERS WHO WILL HELP
US GREET YOU TO HOLD YOU.

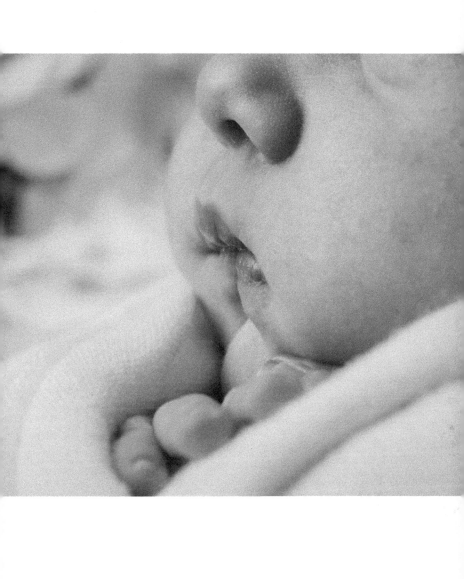

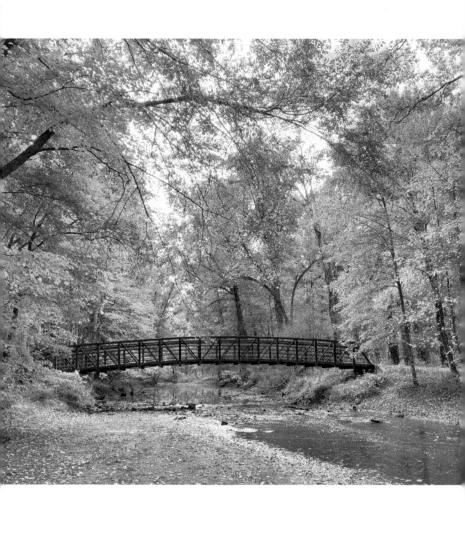

WE ASK OUR HEALED CONSCIOUSNESS TO HOLD YOU.

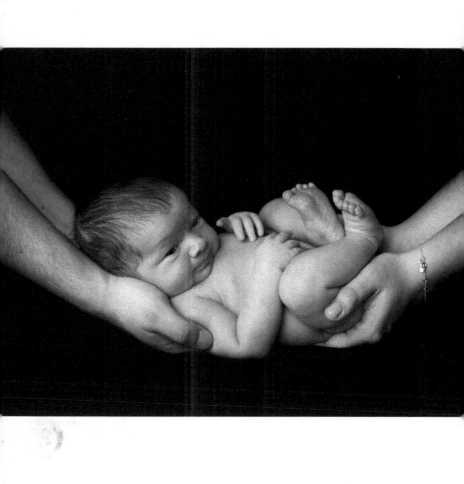

Holding at Birth and Beyond

Dearest Little One,

We are so glad that you are here sweet soul. We are over-joyed to meet you. You are so wanted. You arrived at the perfect time. May you feel our sacred holding in many ways, from the still cadence of our words to the tender scoops into our arms. May you feel embraced with affirmations of love. We hope that you find words one day to tell us how you would like to be held. We hope to hold you in a multitude of ways all the days of your life.

Please know that we will honor you throughout your life by asking, "How would you like to be held?"

WE WELCOME YOU,
HOLDING YOU
WITH OUR GAZE.

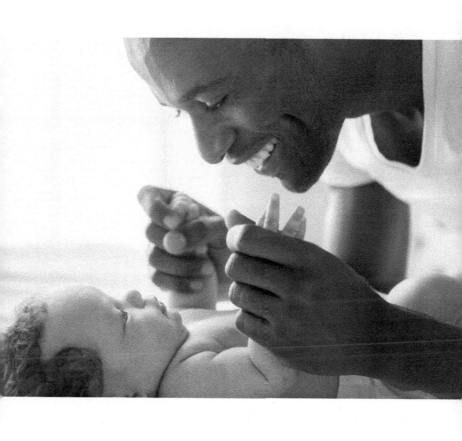

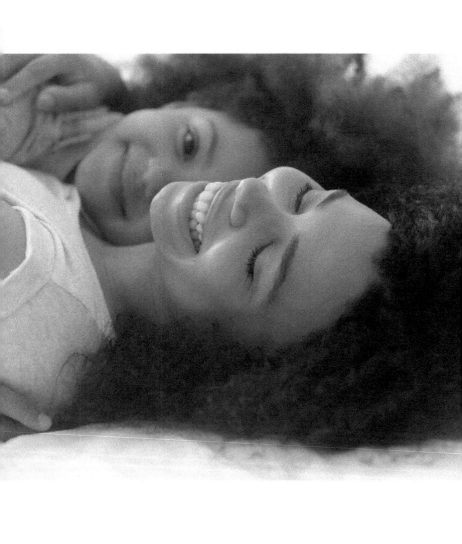

WE WELCOME YOU,
HOLDING YOU
WITH OUR ARMS.

WE WELCOME YOU,
HOLDING YOU
WITH OUR HEARTBEAT.

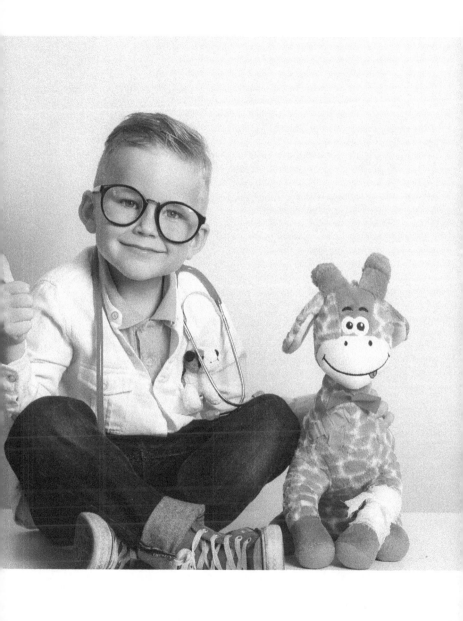

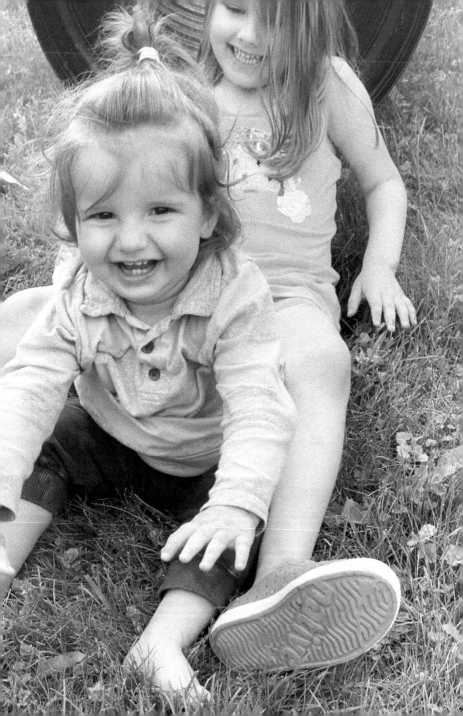

WE WELCOME YOU,
HOLDING YOU
WITH OUR PRESENCE.

WE WELCOME YOU,
HOLDING YOU WITH
THE WALLS OF OUR HOME.

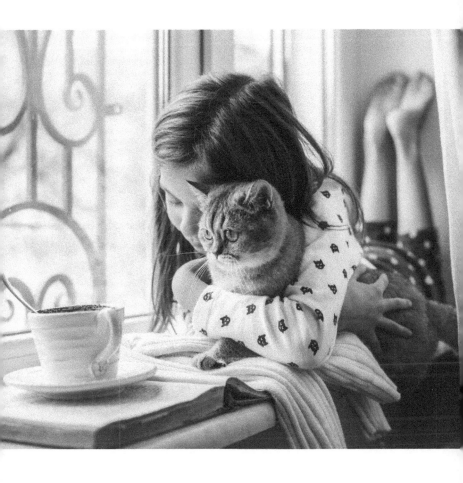

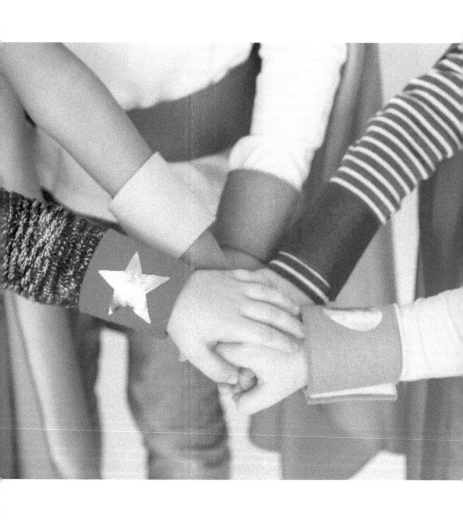

WE WELCOME YOU, HOLDING YOU AND ALL OF YOUR POTENTIALS.

WE WELCOME YOU,
HOLDING YOU
IN SPACIOUSNESS.

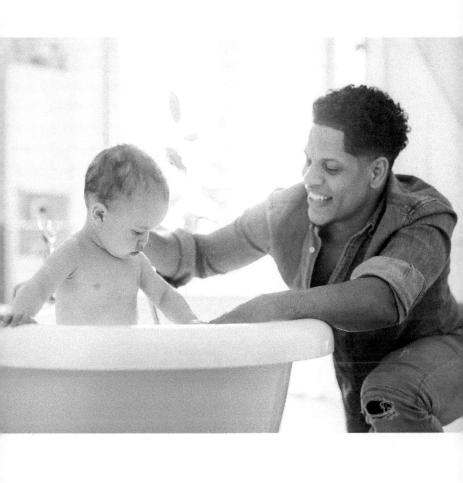

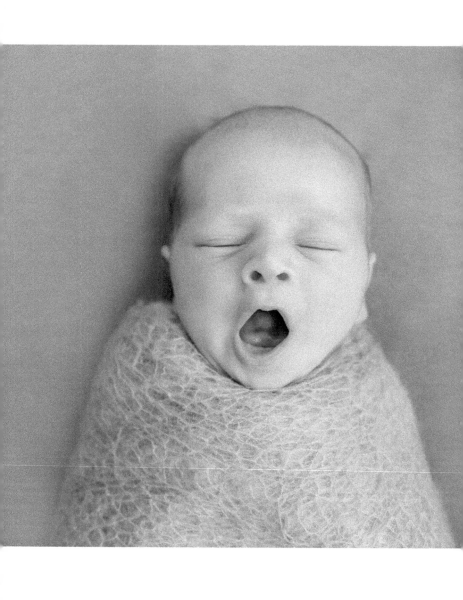

WE WELCOME YOU, HOLDING THE SENTIENCE THAT YOU ARE.

WE WELCOME YOU
WITH SONG.

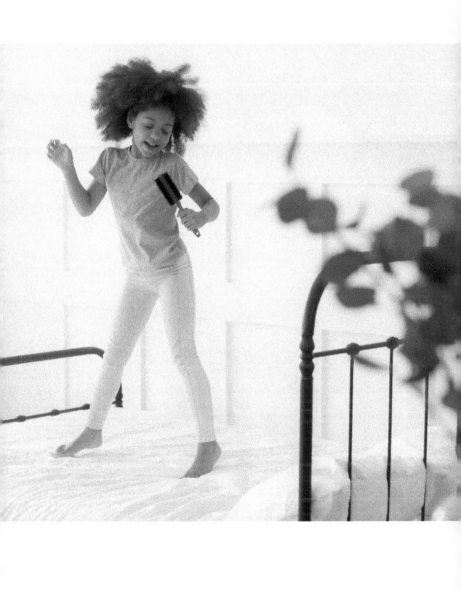

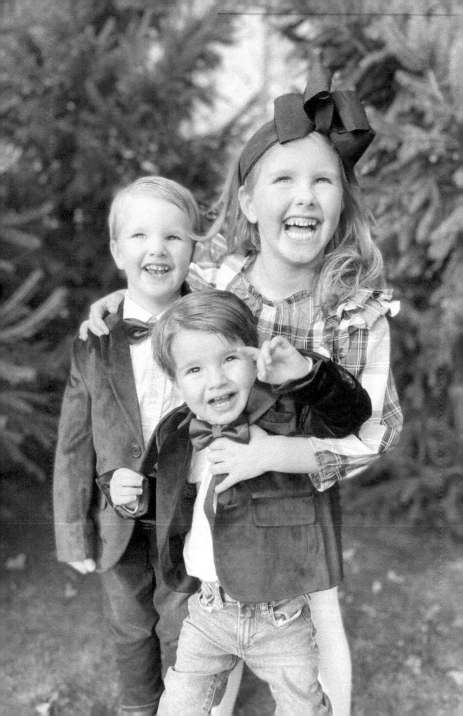

WE WELCOME YOU WITH JOY.

WE WELCOME YOU
WITH SILENCE.

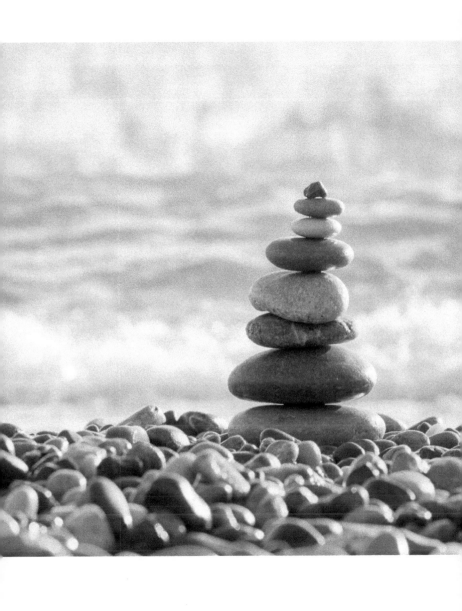

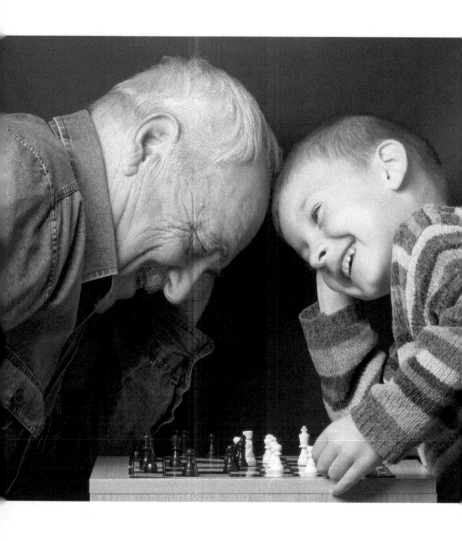

WE WELCOME YOU
WITH WORDS.

WE WELCOME YOU
WITH TENDER TOUCH.

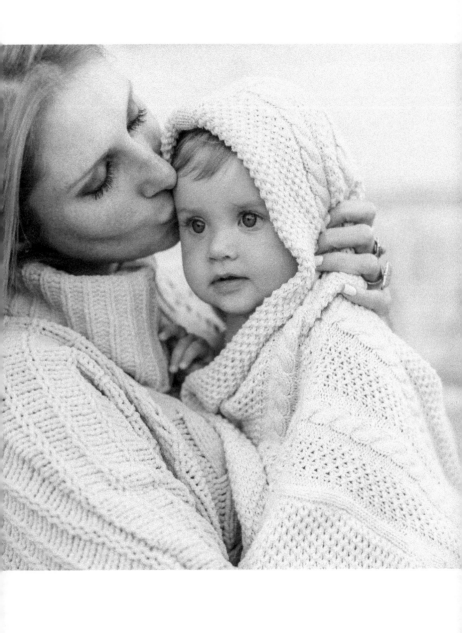

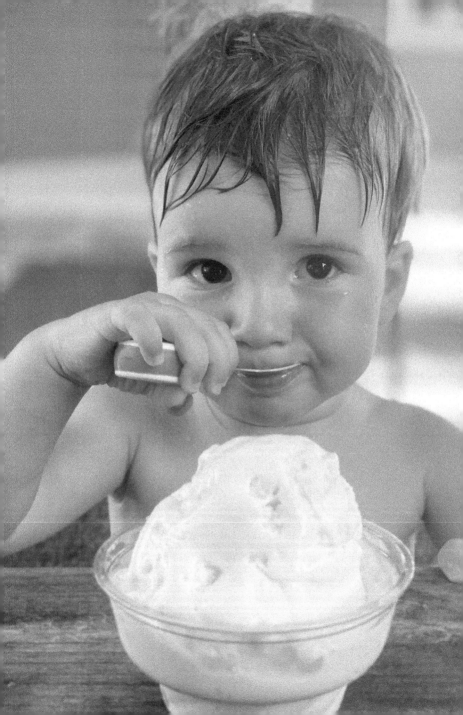

WE WELCOME YOU
WITH OUR HEARTS
WIDE OPEN.

WE WELCOME YOU
WITH CONSCIOUSNESS.

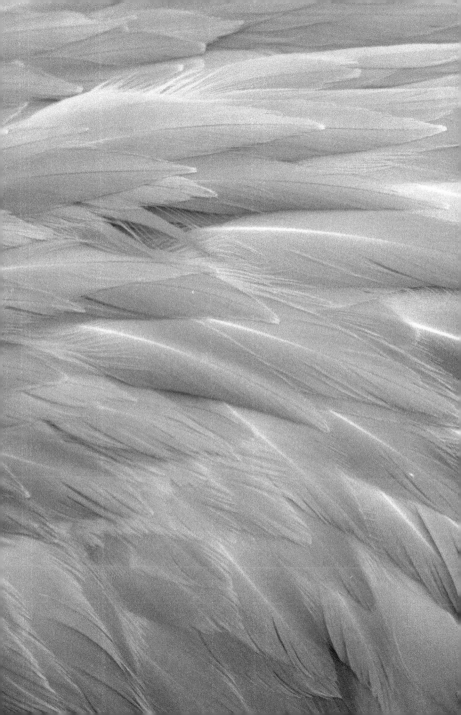

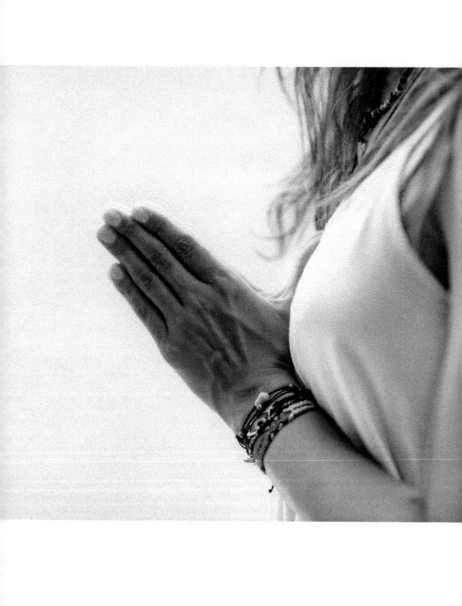

Dearest Parents and Caregivers,

We deeply honor that holding may have been missed in
your history. We take a deep breath with you and offer
that by sharing this conscious gesture of holding with
your baby, you too are receiving a healing and creating
a new way of holding yourself. May you lean into new
ways of care. May you have the audacity to ask others
to embrace you in unique ways. May you also hold
yourself in a new manner.

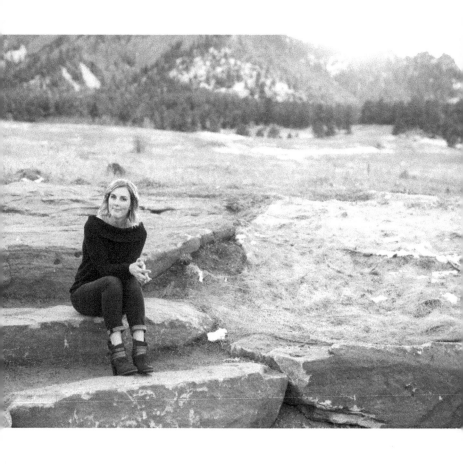

Sarah L. Dickey

Sarah deeply loves spirituality, curiosity, children, books, nature, rituals, astrology, wonder, and a good cuppa coffee. Her work has led to her role as a soul doula, an APPPAH trained Pre and Perinatal Educator, and a Certified Calm Birth Teacher, who works with mommas, families, and groups to rethink and reclaim the birth experience.

Holding is a very personal work as Sarah believes in the power of conscious embrace through every stage of life from preconception and beyond.

Connect with Sarah, her work and service offerings at sarahldickey.com.

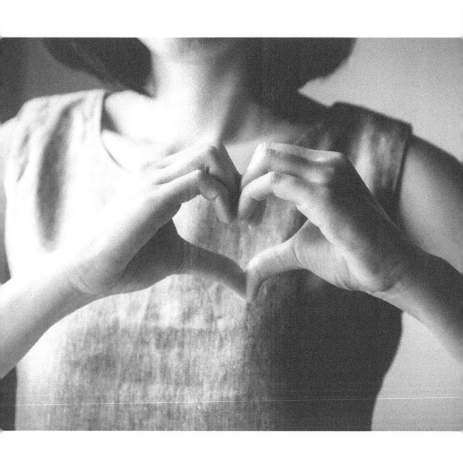

Acknowledgments

Holding was brought to life by many hearts.

Gratitude to my parents, Robert and Nancy who conceived me, and held me for nine months, and who have continued to cheer me on and hold me throughout my life. Thank you. I love you.

Gratitude to my niece and nephews. I love you with all my heart.

Gratitude to all of the wonderful Pre and Perinatal trailblazers who have helped me awaken to the importance of this work, who have helped me to differentiate my history, and create more coherence in my present-day life. There are so many innovative shoulders I am standing upon. I am eternally grateful for your pioneering ways.

Gratitude to my book Sherpa and friend, Gail Kearns of To Press and Beyond, for her unending guidance and expertise as I birth another book into the world. It's always a delight to work with you my dear friend.

Shouts of joy for Cindy Conger, of JustWrite Communications, who has so willingly supported my mission and vision for this book. She has been a midwife championing and encouraging me in my new vision. Thank you to the moon and back for your kindness and impeccable editing.

Alan and Ian of theBookDesigners, your book design talents never cease to amaze me. Thank you again for capturing and bringing to life another offering of my heart.

A huge thank you to Mia Kalef, author of *It's Never Too Late: Healing Prebirth and Birth at Any Age*, and *The Secret Life of Babies: How Our Prebirth and Birth Experiences Shape Our World*, who introduced the concept of a "healed radiant ancestor." Our work together has been life-giving.

Gratitude to Robert Newman and his extraordinary team of hearts at Calm Birth. Calm Birth is a tool of consciousness to support pregnancy and literally every breath of life. I am so grateful for your life-giving work.

Huge gratitude to a dear mentor, Ray Castellino, who literally changed my life and way forward in the world. Thank you for holding such sacred space in my womb surround and teachings that I could know an even greater way of showing up in my life. I love you.

To my dear friend, mentor and spiritual coach, Tom Gigliotti, thank you for all the ways you have held me over the years as I have worked to make the unconscious conscious. I am ever grateful for you. I love you, compadre!

To all of my teachers, from the natural world to the physical flesh. I honor you and am so grateful for your compassion and love.

To my family, thank you for love, support and encouragement. You are delights to me!

To my community and friends, I see you. Your support and love have helped me to build potency in my passion and offerings in the world. I just love you!

To the babies entering our world at this time, I am sending you ALL so much love! Welcome sweet souls. It is an honor to celebrate your presence on our Earth. I pray that you experience unlimited love and deep holding in your lives.

And to everyone reading this, may you feel held. May you explore your life with curiosity, and may you welcome yourself in a whole new way.

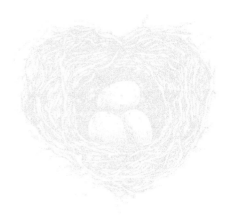